NOSTALGIAWORKS
COMPANION READING

COPYRIGHT AND PERMISSIONS NOTICE

For partnership inquiries, bulk orders, institutional sales, or permissions request, contact NostalgiaWorks at info@nostalgiaworks.com or visit nostalgiaworks.com

NANA'S BOOKS, a Connecticut Limited Liability Company,
DBA NostalgiaWorks

nostalgiaworks.com

Dedication

For the Steady Ground Beneath Our Feet

This collection is compiled with profound gratitude for our caregivers, whose patience stretches wider than the sea, and for our elders, whose light remains a constant blessing
in this world.

Though the landscape around us may change, the roots of our shared love, our deep heritage, and our ancestral quiet stay forever unbroken.

Cover Art:
Winslow Homer, *Native Hut at Nassau*, 1885

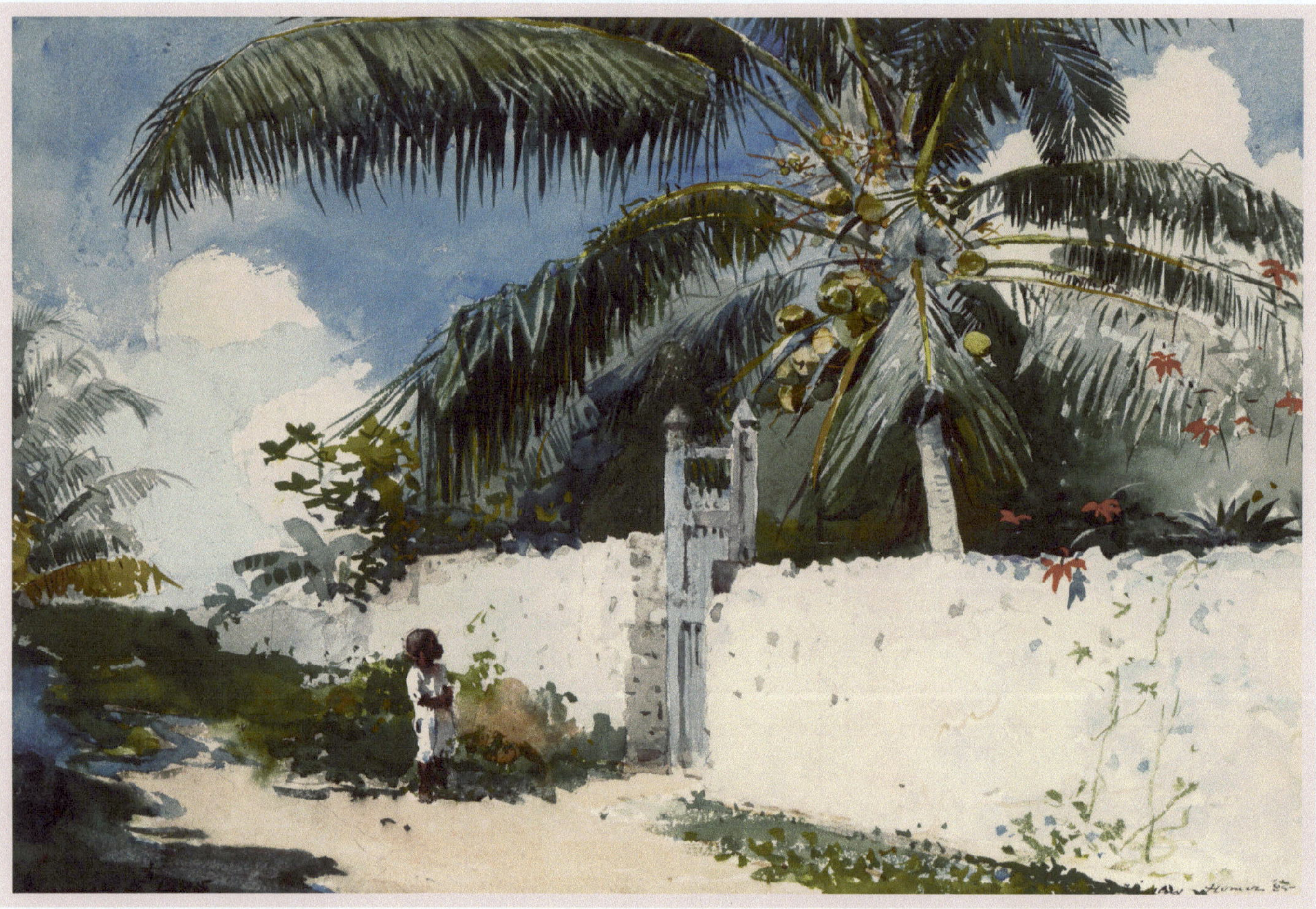

Winslow Homer, *A Garden in Nassau*, 1885

The Easter Flower

Far from this foreign Easter damp and chilly
My soul steals to a pear-shaped plot of ground,
Where gleamed the lilac-tinted Easter lily
Soft-scented in the air for yards around;

Alone, without a hint of guardian leaf!
Just like a fragile bell of silver rime,
It burst the tomb for freedom sweet and brief
In the young pregnant year at Eastertime;

And many thought it was a sacred sign,
And some called it the resurrection flower;
And I, a pagan, worshiped at its shrine,
Yielding my heart unto its perfumed power.

Claude McKay, 1920

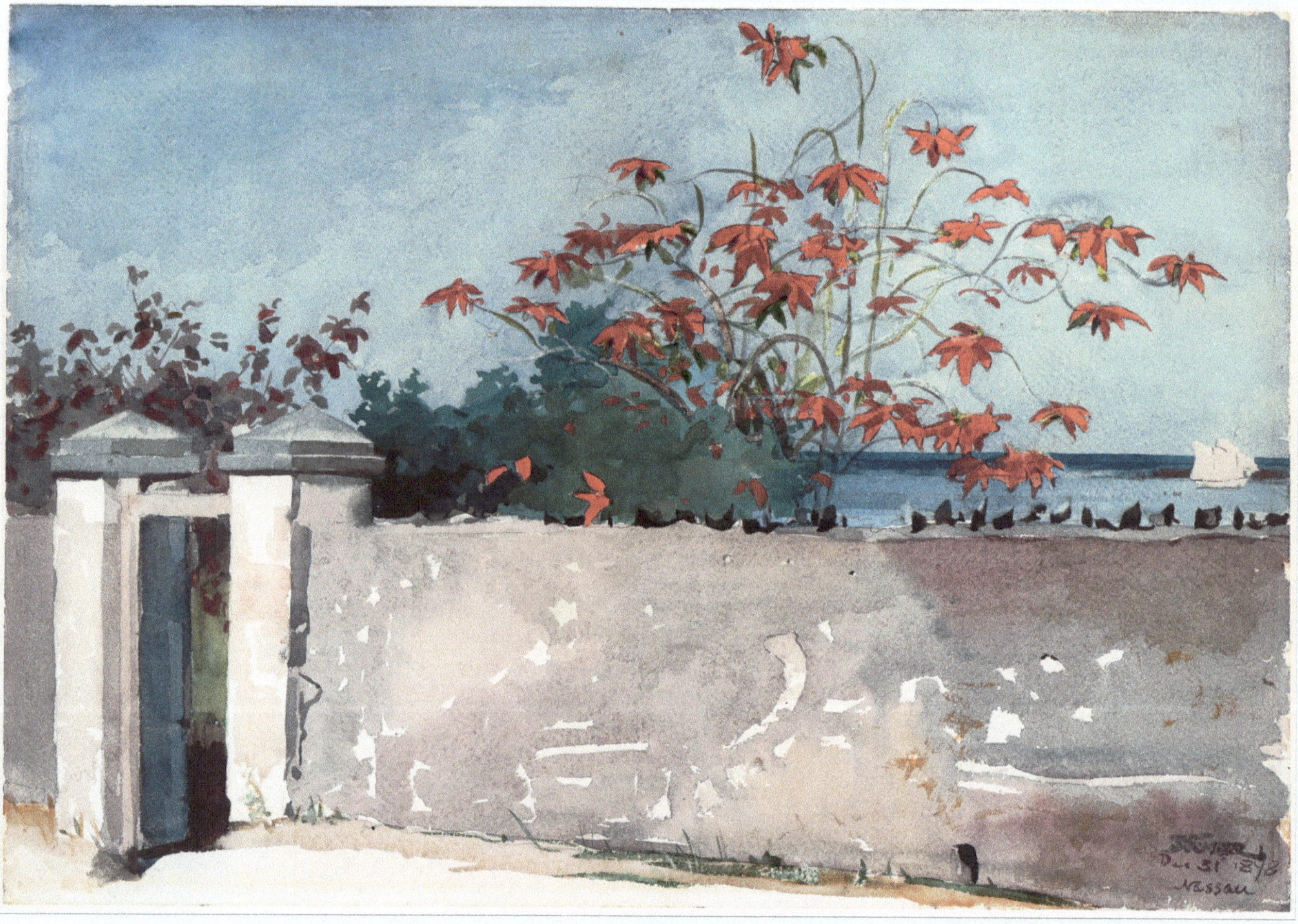

Winslow Homer, A Wall, Nassau, 1898

Morning Star

Morning Star, O cheering sight!
Ere thou camest how dark earth's night!
Morning Star, O cheering sight!
Ere thou camest how dark earth's night!

Jesus mine,
in me shine;
In me shine,
Jesus mine.
Fill my heart with light divine.

Morning Star, thy glory bright
far excels the sun's clear light.
Morning Star, thy glory bright
far excels the sun's clear light.
Jesus be,
constantly,
constantly,
constantly,
more than a thousand suns to me.

Moravian Hymn, Traditional

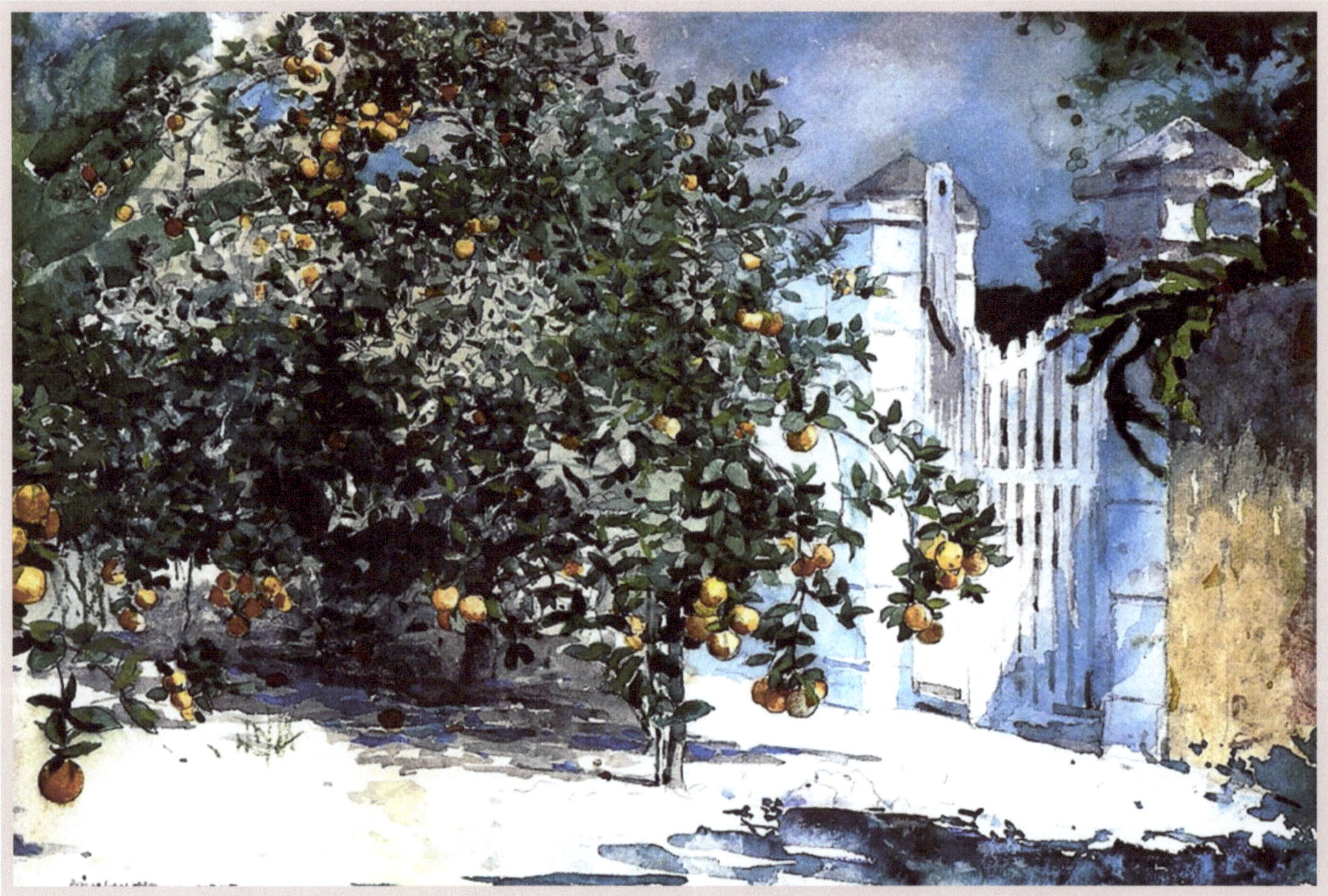

Winslow Homer, *Orange Tree,* Nassau, 1885

The Tropics in New York

Bananas ripe and green, and ginger-root,
Cocoa in pods and alligator pears,
And tangerines and mangoes and grapefruit,
Fit for the highest prize at parish fairs,

Set in the window, bringing memories
Of fruit-trees laden by the low-singing rills,
And dewy dawns, and mystical blue skies
In benediction o'er the nun-like hills.

My eyes grew dim, and I could no more gaze;
A wave of longing shut my sight from view,
And, hungry for the old, familiar ways,
I turned aside and bowed my head and wept.

Claude McKay, 1920

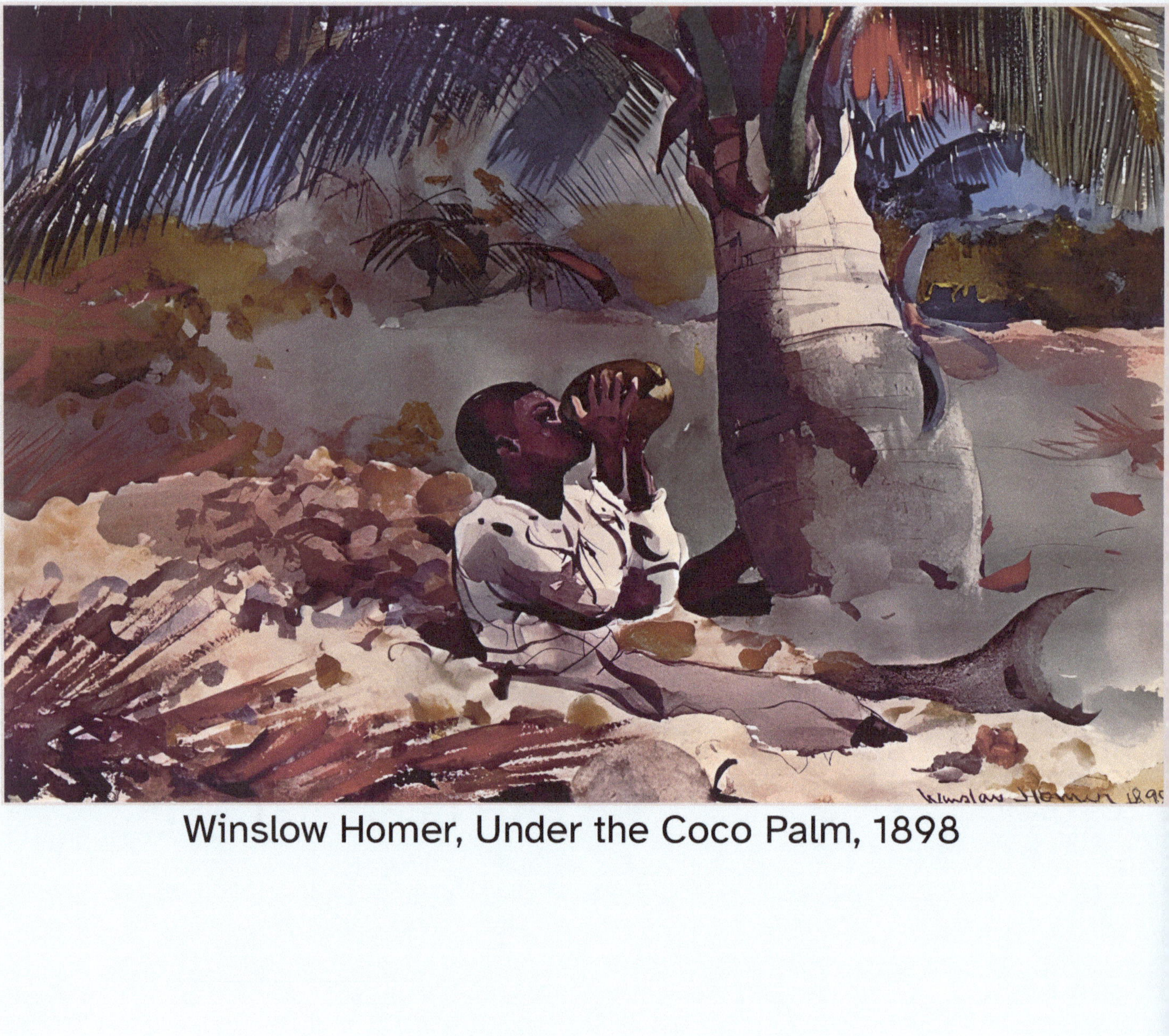

Winslow Homer, Under the Coco Palm, 1898

Flame Heart

So much have I forgotten in ten years,
So much in ten brief years; I have forgot
What time the purple apples come to juice
And what month brings the shy forget-me-not;

Forgotten is the special, startling season
Of some beloved tree's flowering and fruiting,
What time of year the ground doves brown the fields
And fill the noonday with their curious fluting:

I have forgotten much, but still remember
The poinsettia's red, blood-red in warm December.

I still recall the honey-fever grass,
But I cannot bring back to mind just when
We rooted them out of the ping-wing path
To stop the mad bees in the rabbit pen.

I often try to think in what sweet month
The languid painted ladies used to dapple
The yellow bye road mazing from the main,
Sweet with the golden threads of the rose-apple:

I have forgotten, strange, but quite remember
The poinsettia's red, blood-red in warm December.

Claude McKay, 1920

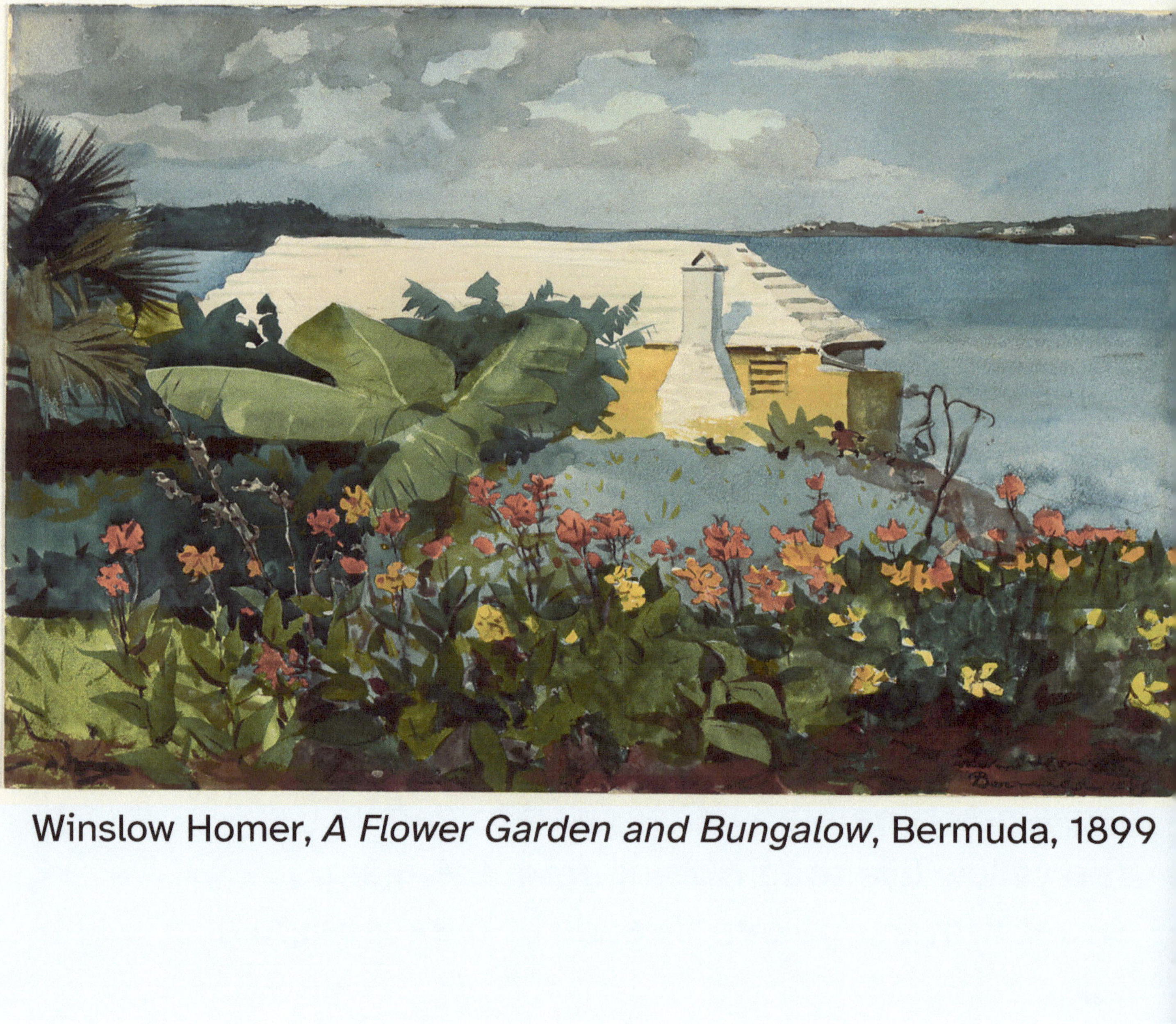

Winslow Homer, *A Flower Garden and Bungalow*, Bermuda, 1899

Spanish Needle

Lovely dainty Spanish needle
With your yellow flower and white,
Dew bedecked and softly sleeping,
Do you think of me to-night?
Shadowed by the spreading mango,
Nodding o'er the rippling stream,
Tell me, dear plant of my childhood,
Do you of the exile dream?
Do you see me by the brook's side
Catching crayfish 'neath the stone,
As you did the day you whispered:
Leave the harmless dears alone?
Do you see me in the meadow
Coming from the woodland spring
With a bamboo on my shoulder
And a pail sling from a string?
Do you see me all expectant
Lying in an orange grove,
While the swee-swees sing above me,
Waiting for my elf-eyed love?
Lovely dainty Spanish needle,
Source to me of sweet delight,
In your far-off sunny southland
Do you dream of me to-night?

Claude McKay, 1922

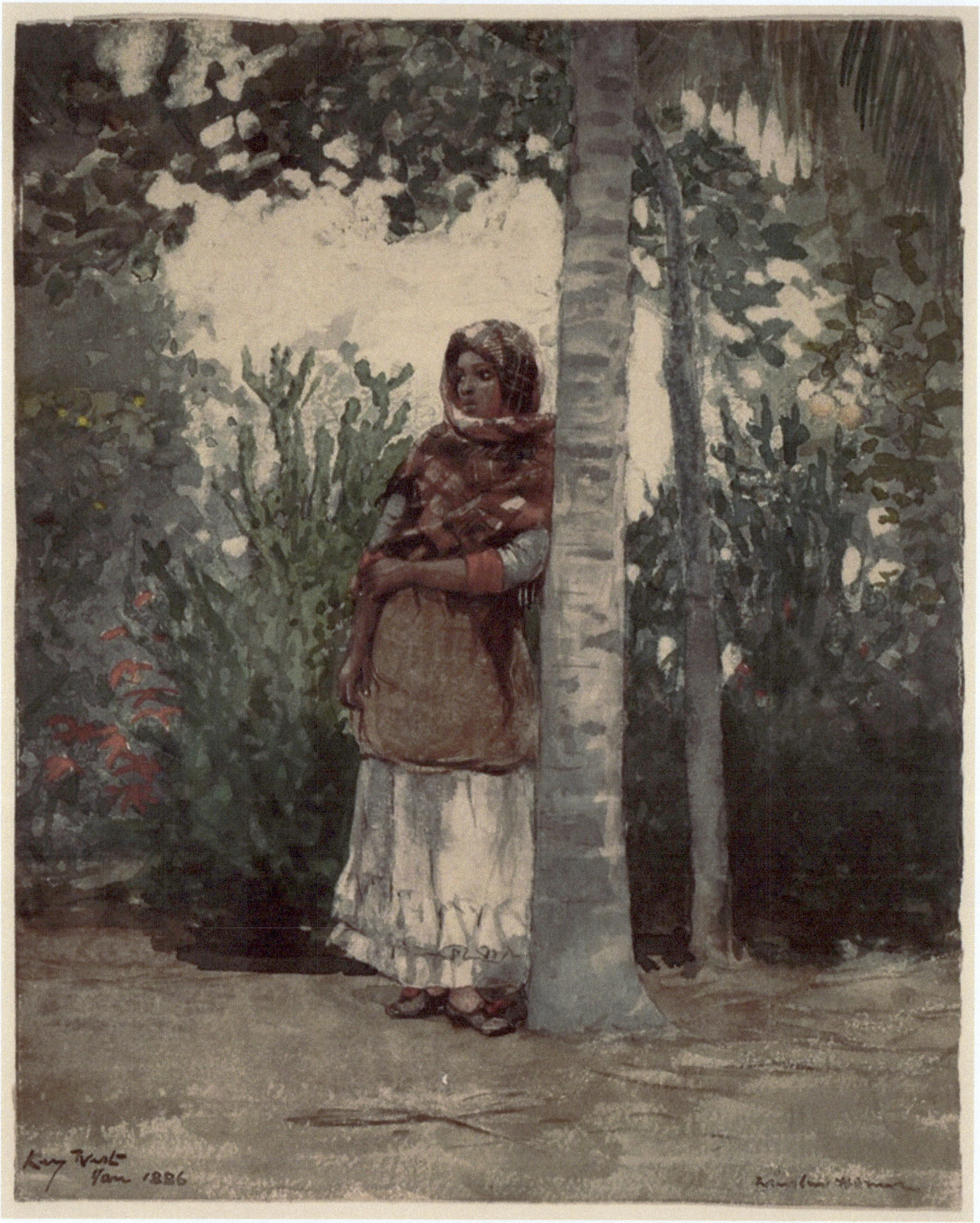

Winslow Homer, *Under a Palm Tree*, 1886

I Shall Return

I shall return again; I shall return
To laugh and love and watch with wonder-eyes
At golden noon the forest fires burn,
Wafting their blue-black smoke to sapphire skies.

I shall return to loiter by the streams
That bathe the brown blades of the bending grasses,
And realize once more my thousand dreams
Of waters rushing down the mountain passes.

I shall return to hear the fiddle and fife
Of village dances, dear delicious tunes
That stir the hidden depths of native life,
Stray melodies of dim remembered runes.

I shall return, I shall return again,
To ease my mind of long, long years of pain.

Claude McKay, 1920

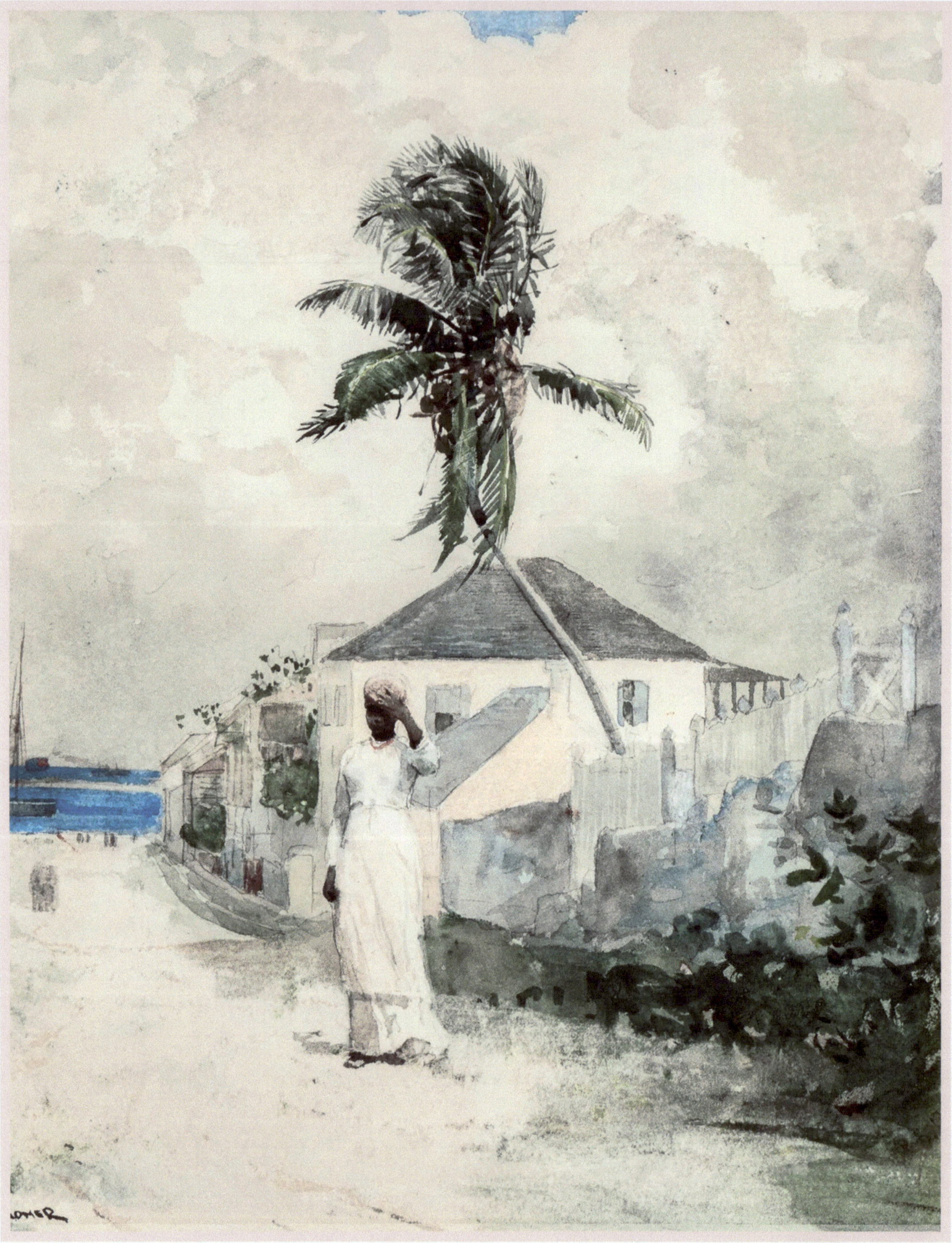

Winslow Homer, *Along the Road, Bahamas,* 1885

However far the stream flows,
it never forgets its source.
— African proverb

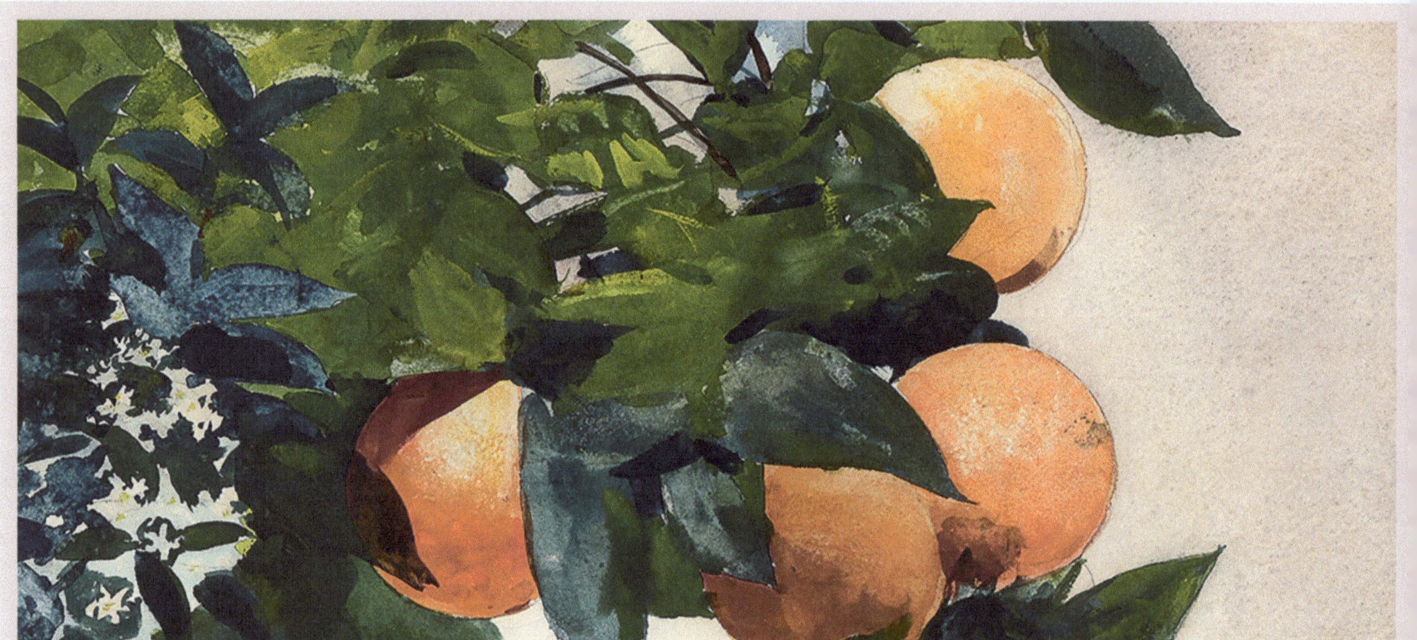

Winslow Homer, *Oranges on a Branch*, 1885

After the Winter

Some day, when trees have shed their leaves
And against the morning's white
The shivering birds beneath the eaves
Have sheltered for the night,

We'll turn our faces southward, love,
Toward the summer isle
Where bamboos spire to shafted grove
And wide-mouthed orchids smile.

And we will seek the quiet hill
Where towers the cotton tree,
And leaps the laughing crystal rill,
And works the droning bee.

And we will build a cottage there
Beside an open glade,
With black-ribbed blue-bells blowing near,
And ferns that never fade.

Claude McKay, 1920

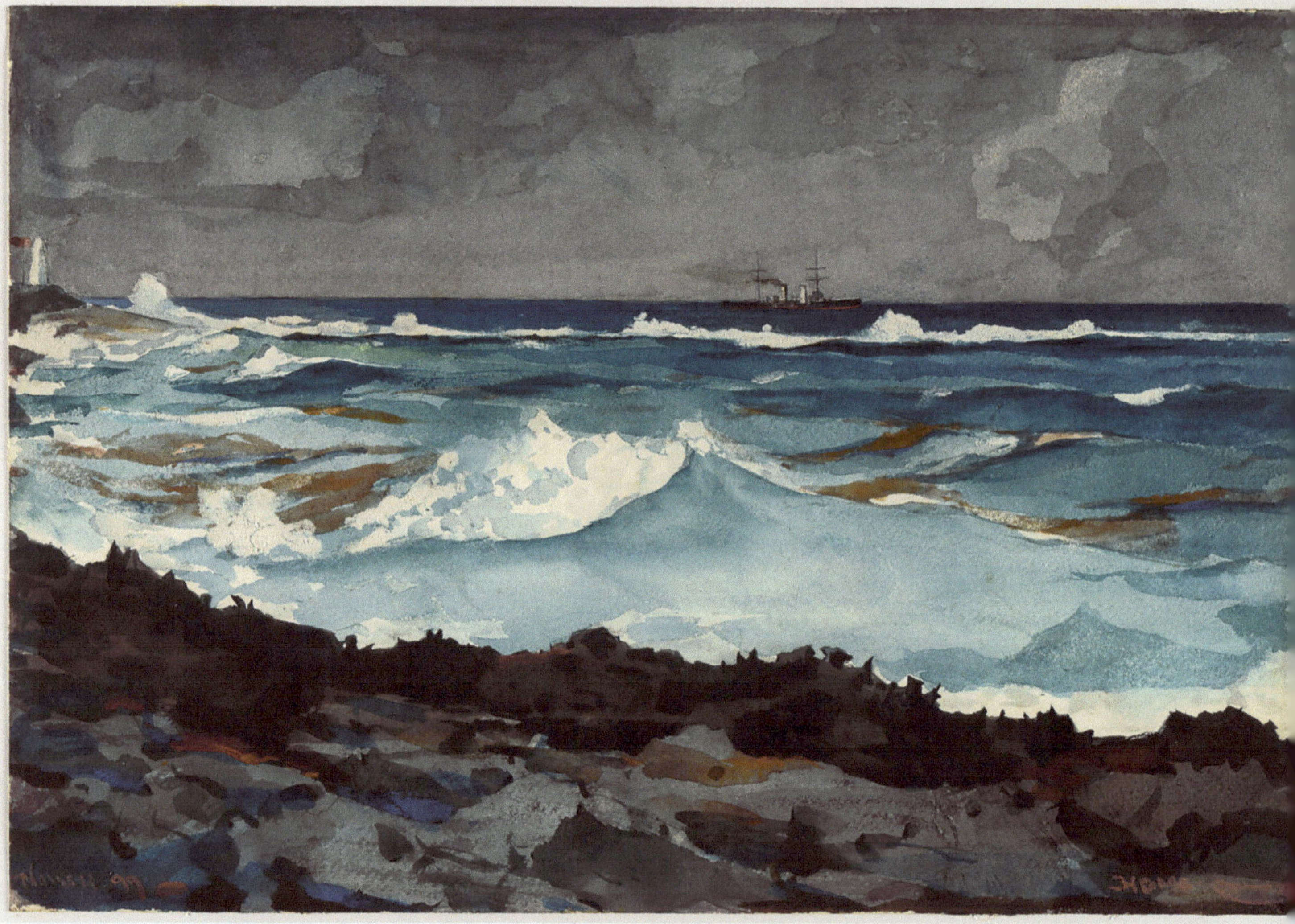

Winslow Homer, *Shore and Surf*, Nassau 1885

However long the night,
the dawn will break.

-African Proverb

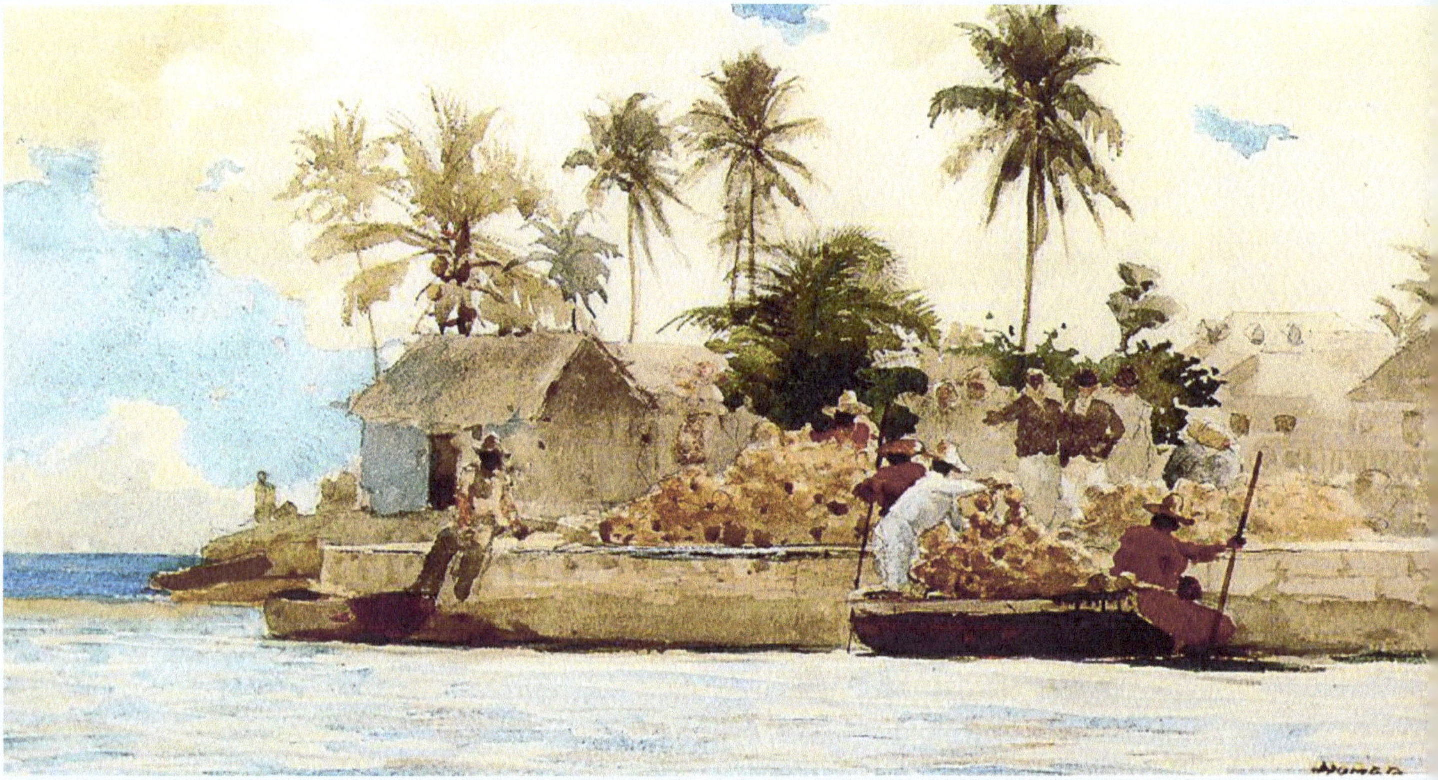

Winslow Homer, Sponge Fishermen, Bahamas, 1885

The Aaronic Blessing

God bless you and keep you.

God smile on you and gift you.

God look you full in the face and make you prosper.

King James Bible, Numbers, 6:24–26

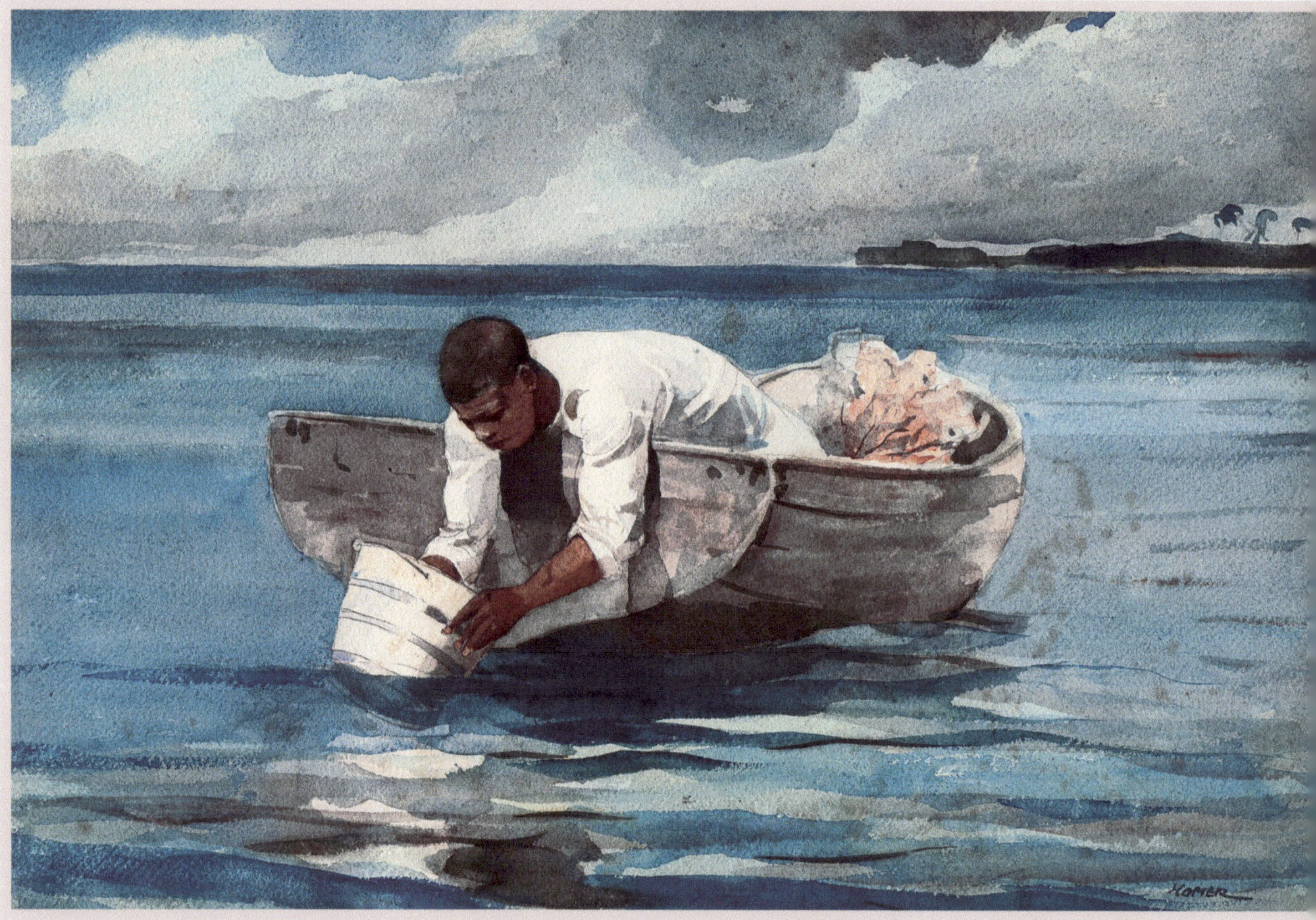

Winslow Homer, *The Water Fan*, 1898

Eternal Father, Strong to Save

Eternal Father, strong to save,
Whose arm does bind the restless wave,
Who bids the mighty ocean deep
Its own appointed limits keep;

O hear us when we cry to Thee
For those in peril on the sea.
O Savior, whose almighty word
The winds and waves submissive heard,

Who walked upon the foaming deep,
And calm amid the rage did sleep;
O hear us when we cry to Thee
For those in peril on the sea.

O Holy Spirit, who did brood
Upon the waters dark and rude,
And bid their angry tumult cease,
And give for wild confusion peace;

O hear us when we cry to Thee
For those in peril on the sea.
O Trinity of love and pow'r,
Your children shield in danger's hour;

From rock and tempest, fire, and foe,
Protect them where-so-e'er they go;
Thus, evermore shall rise to Thee Glad

William Whiting 1860

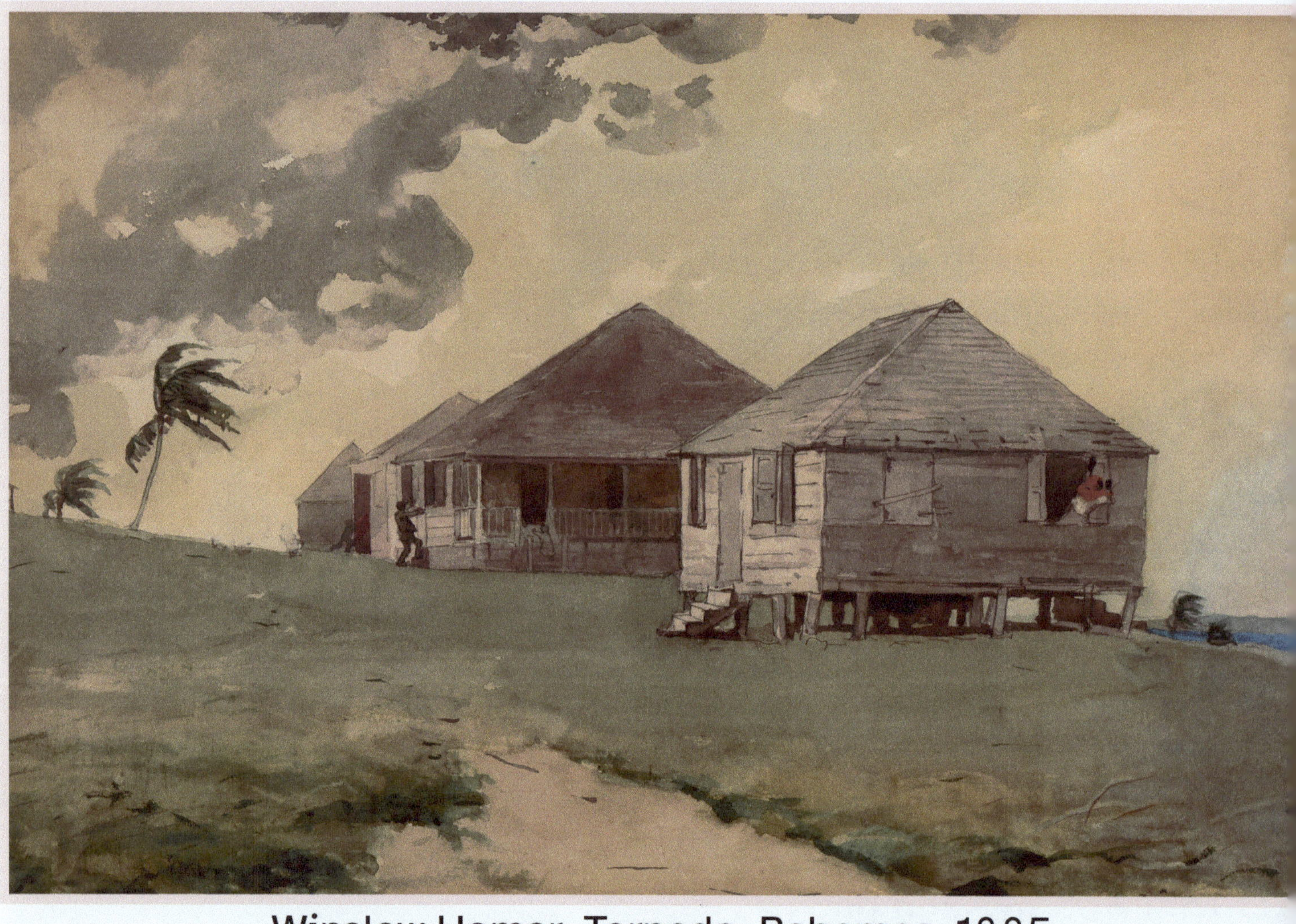

Winslow Homer, Tornado, Bahamas, 1885

What a Friend We Have in Jesus

What a friend we have in Jesus, all our sins and griefs to bear!
What a privilege to carry everything to God in prayer!
O what peace we often forfeit, O what needless pain we bear,
All because we do not carry everything to God in prayer.

Have we trials and temptations? Is there trouble anywhere?
We should never be discouraged; take it to the Lord in prayer.
Can we find a friend so faithful, who will all our sorrows share?
Jesus knows our every weakness; take it to the Lord in prayer.

Are we weak and heavy laden, cumbered with a load of care?
Precious Savior, still our refuge; take it to the Lord in prayer.
Do thy friends despise, forsake thee?
Take it to the Lord in prayer!
In his arms he'll take and shield thee; thou wilt find a solace there.

Joseph Scriven, 1855

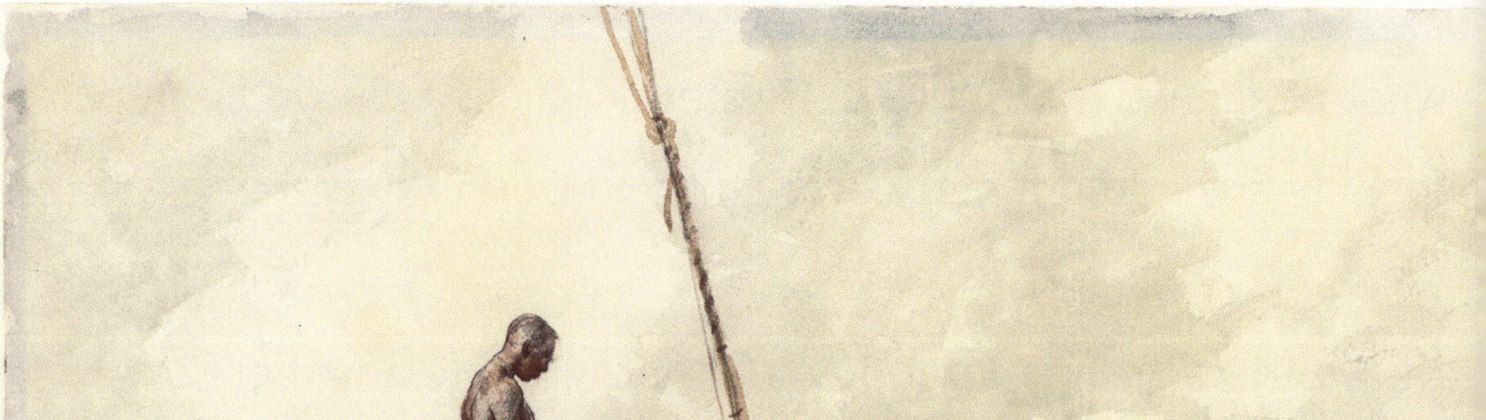

Winslow Homer, The Conch Divers, 1885

Home Thoughts

Oh something just now must be happening there!
That suddenly and quiveringly here,
Amid the city's noises, I must think
Of mangoes leaning o'er the river's brink,

And dexterous Davie climbing high above,
The gold fruits ebon-speckled to remove,
And toss them quickly in the tangled mass
Of wis-wis twisted round the guinea grass;

And Cyril coming through the bramble-track
A prize bunch of bananas on his back;
And Georgie—none could ever dive like him—
Throwing his scanty clothes off for a swim;

And schoolboys, from Bridge-tunnel going home,
Watching the waters downward dash and foam.
This is no daytime dream, there's something in it,
Oh something's happening there this very minute!

Claude McKay, 1920

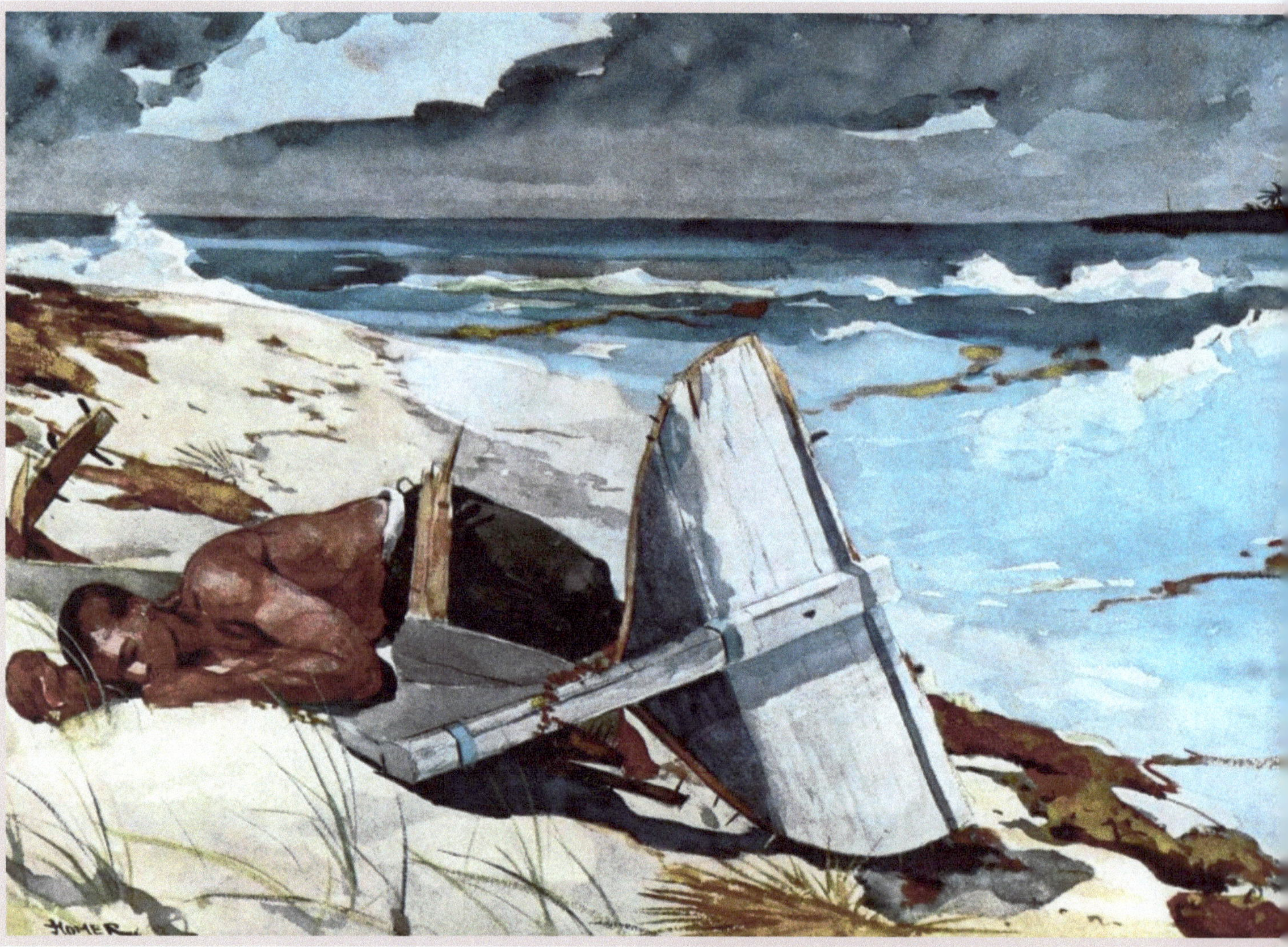

Winslow Homer, After the Hurricane, Bahamas, 1899

The Day is Past and Gone

The day is past and gone,
The evening shades appear;
O may we all remember well
The night of life draws near.
We lay our garments by,
Upon our beds to rest;
So death will soon disrobe us all
Of what we here possessed.
Lord, keep us safe this night,
Secure from all our fears;
May angels guard us while we sleep,
Till morning light appears.

John Leland, 1792

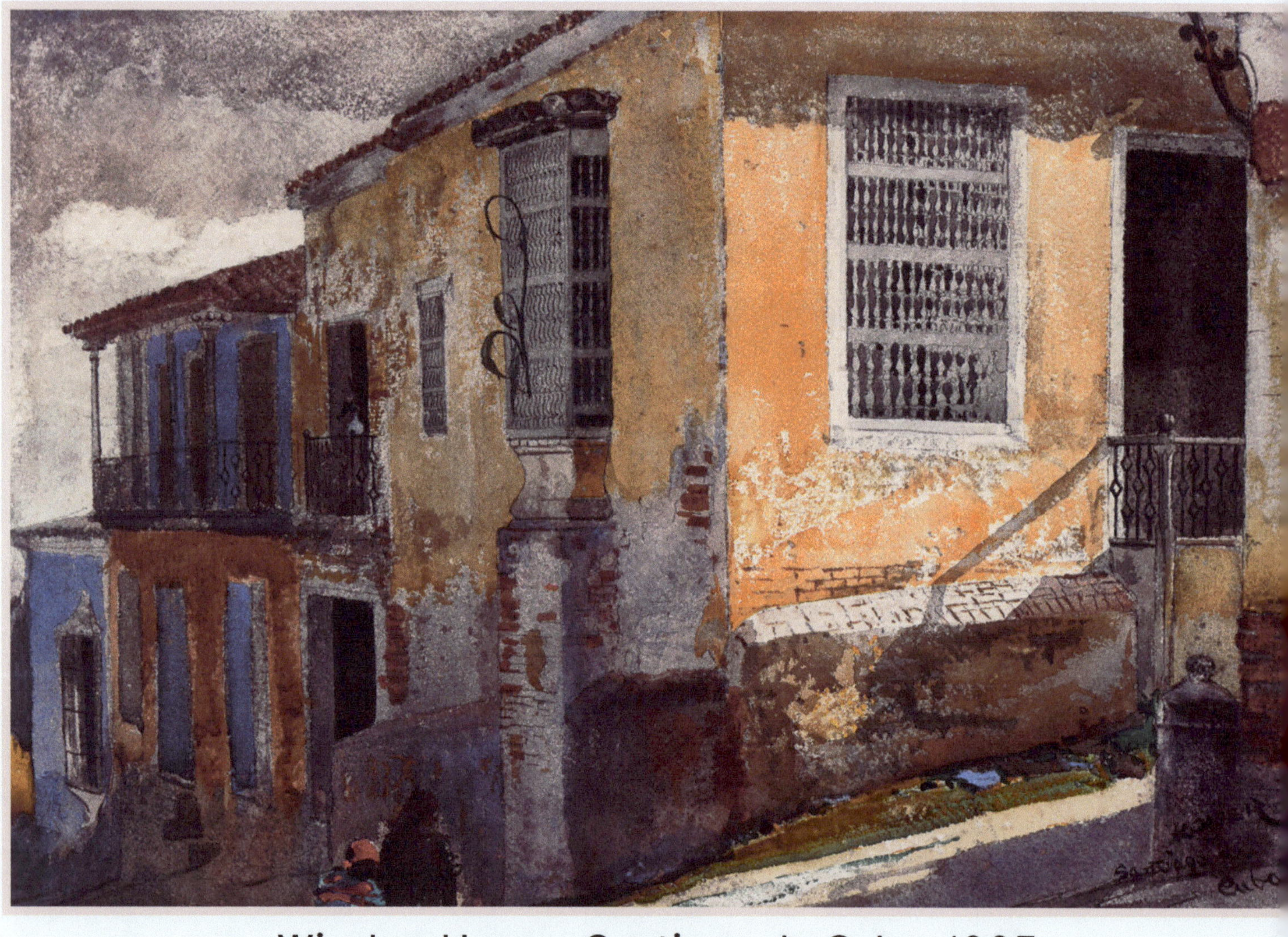

Winslow Homer, Santiago de Cuba, 1885

Sweet and Low

Sweet and low, sweet and low,
Wind of the western sea,
Low, low, breathe and blow,
Wind of the western sea!

Over the rolling waters go,
Come from the dying moon, and blow,
Blow him again to me;
While my little one, while my pretty one, sleeps.

Sleep and rest, sleep and rest,
Father will come to thee soon;
Rest, rest, on mother's breast,
Father will come to thee soon;

Father will come to his babe in the nest,
Silver sails all out of the west
Under the silver moon:
Sleep, my little one, sleep, my pretty one, sleep.

Alfred Lord Tennyson, 1849

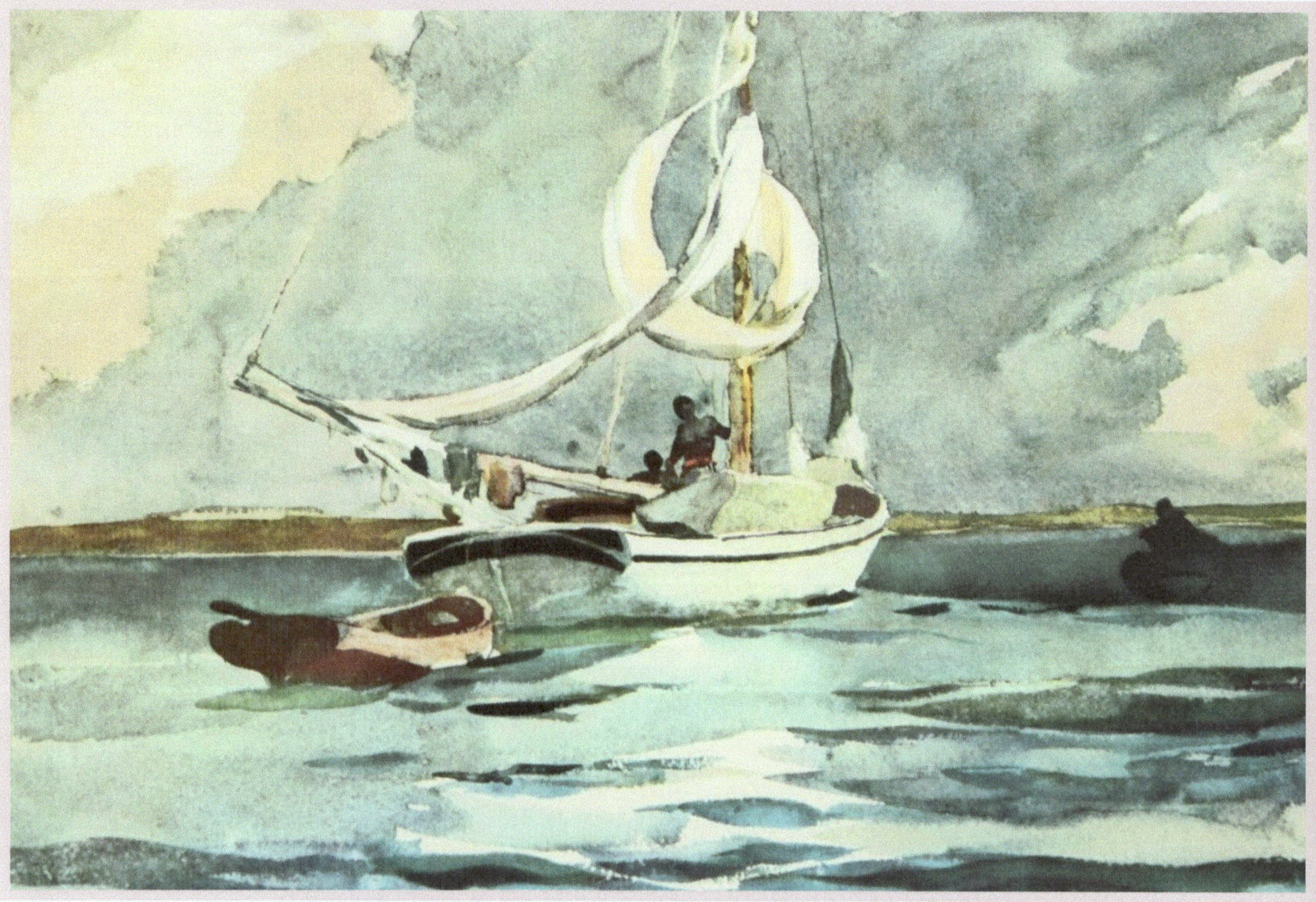

Winslow Homer, *Sloop, Nassau* (1899)

Abide with Me

Abide with me, fast falls the eventide,
The darkness deepens; Lord, with me abide!
When other helpers fail and comforts flee,
Help of the helpless, O abide with me.

Swift to its close ebbs out life's little day,
Earth's joys grow dim, its glories pass away;
Change and decay in all around I see:
O Thou who changest not, abide with me.

I need Thy presence ev'ry passing hour;
What but Thy grace can foil the tempter's pow'r?
Who, like Thyself, my guide and stay can be?
Through cloud and sunshine, O abide with me.

Henry Francis Lyte, 1847

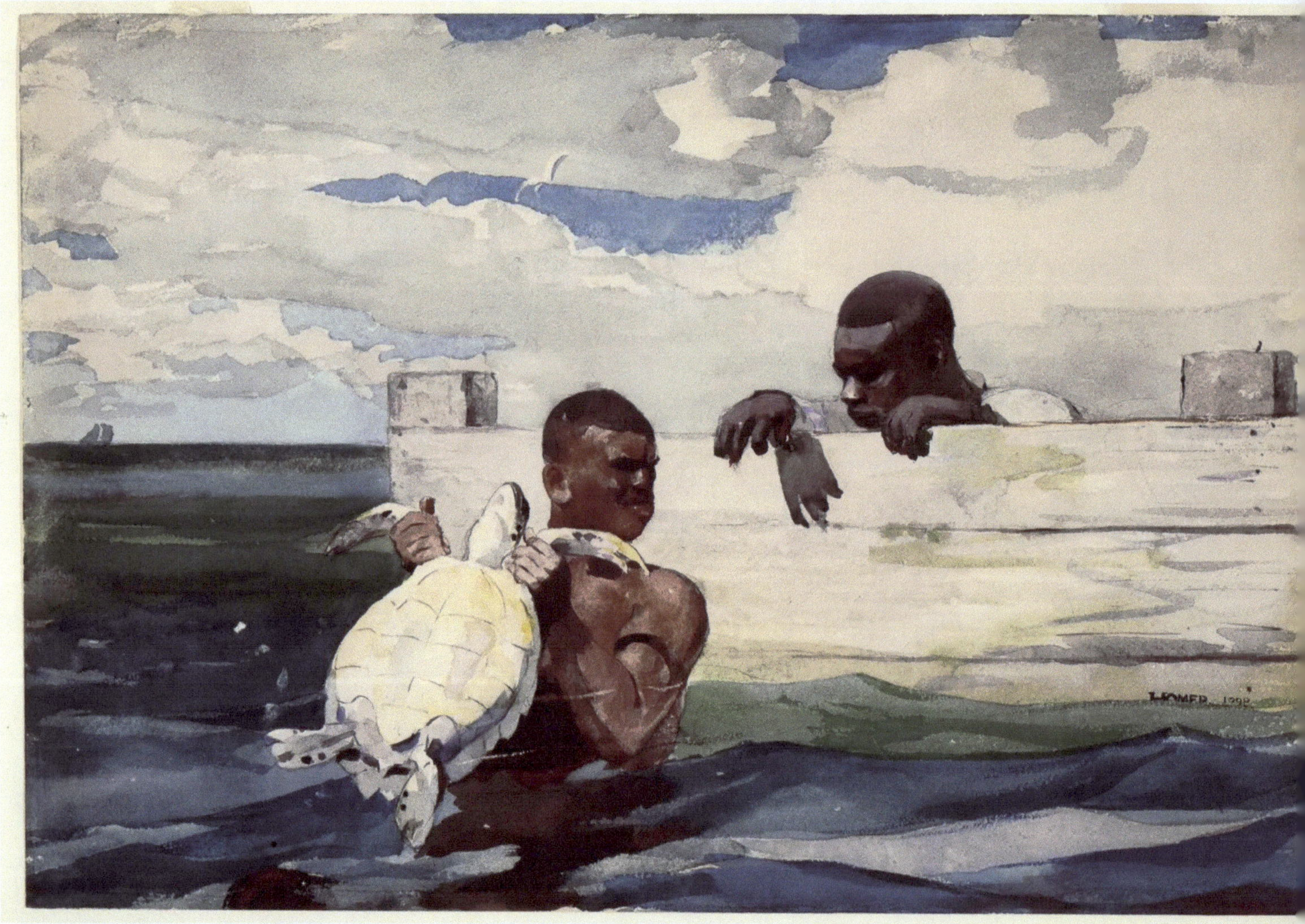

Winslow Homer, *The Turtle Pond*, 1898

On Glory

Now unto him that is able to keep you from falling,

and to present you faultless

before the presence of His glory

with exceeding joy,

to the only wise God our Saviour,

beglory and majesty,

dominion and power,

both now and ever.

Amen.

Jude 1:24-25, King James Bible

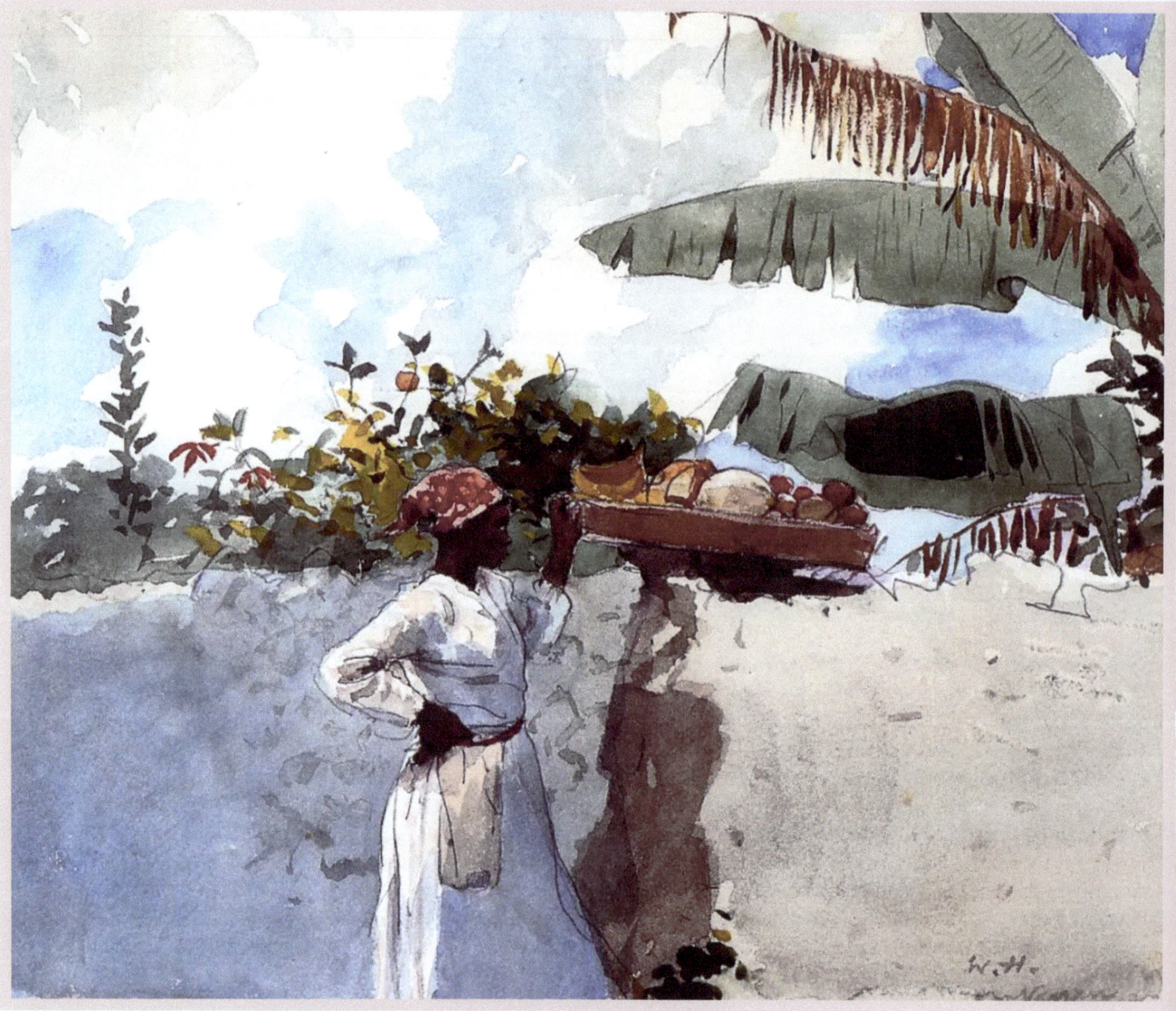

Winslow Homer, *Rest*, 1885

BOOK CHAT

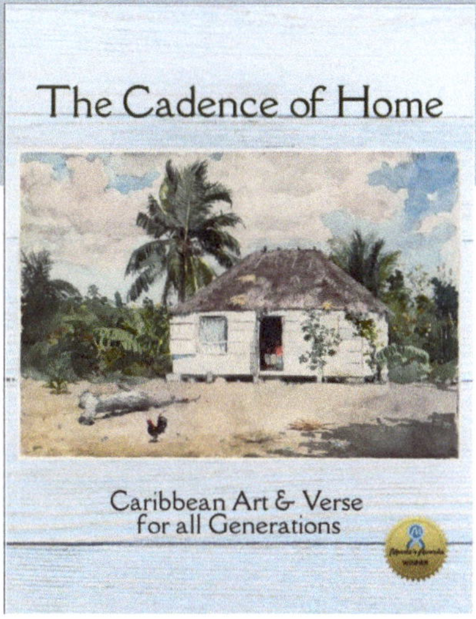

LET'S FIND...

- A thatched-roof cottage
- Chickens in the yard
- A sloop with white sails
- An orange tree heavy with fruit
- Red flowers climbing an old wall
- Sponge fishermen at work
- Palm trees bending in the wind

FUN FACTS!

-Claude McKay grew up in the hills of Clarendon Parish, Jamaica, and wrote his earliest poems about the plants, brooks, and fruit trees of his childhood before ever leaving the island.

-"Mi navel string bury deh" is a Jamaican saying meaning "my navel string is buried there" is a tradition of burying a newborn's umbilical cord under a young tree, binding the child to home soil for life.

-Mangoes, tamarind, and breadfruit all traveled to the Caribbean by ship; breadfruit famously arriving from the South Pacific in 1793, and became beloved staples of island life.

AUTHOR SHARE:

I recall two incredible trips to Barbados when our children were small. We stayed on the southwest side of the Island and the winds were fierce. One day, when the sea was quiet, I watched my husband and three children swim with the leatherback turtles. What a moment of pure joy. Have you ever had an unforgettable brush with nature like we did?

www.ingramcontent.com/pod-product-compliance
Lightning Source LLC
LaVergne TN
LVHW070627061126
851857LV00003B/31